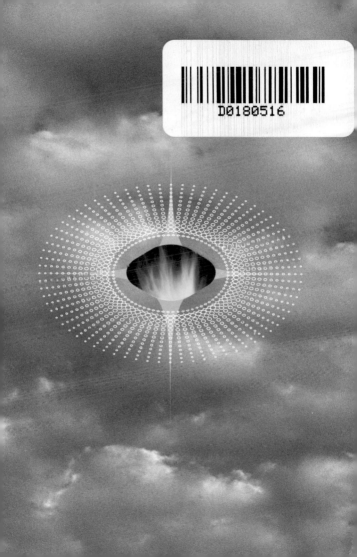

LIFT ME UP

Stephanie Tourles

REVITALIZE, ENERGIZE, AND INVIGORATE YOUR BODY & MIND

The mission of Storey Publishing is to serve our customers by publishing practical information that encourages personal independence in harmony with the environment.

Edited by Deborah Balmuth and Carey L. Boucher
Art direction by Joshua C. Chen and Cindy McFarland
Book design and illustrations by Chen Design Associates

The information in this book is true and complete to the best of our knowledge. All recommendations are made without guarantee on the part of the author or Storey Publishing. The author and publisher disclaim any liability in connection with the use of this information. For additional information please contact Storey Publishing, 210 MASS MoCA Way, North Adams, MA 01247.

Storey books are available for special premium and promotional uses and for customized editions. For further information, please call 1-800-793-9396.

Printed in Hong Kong by Elegance
10 9 8 7 6 5 4 3 2 1

Library of Congress Cataloging-in-Publication Data
Tourles, Stephanie.
  Lift me up, calm me down / by Stephanie Tourles and Barbara L. Heller.
       p. cm.
  ISBN 1-58017-163-X (alk. paper)
  1. Health. 2. Vitality. 3. Stress management. I. Tourles, Stephanie L. 1962- II. Title.

RA776.T7263 2003
613—dc21   2003050559

To Nancy —

A truly natural beauty.

An artistic and creative soul.

Fastest glue gun in the East.

Forever 39.

Thanks for valuing the colors, textures, and scents nature has to offer and sharing that knowledge with me. You're the best mother-in-law a girl could ask for.

Acknowledgments

My heartfelt appreciation goes out to the many who have shared their personal solutions and secrets for revitalizing, re-energizing, and restoring their bodies, minds, and spirits in these busy and trying times. Thanks so much for your ideas and inspiration.

Are you in need of a lift? An energetic boost? If so, you're not alone. Lack of energy, be it physical or mental, is the most common health complaint today.

Energy…what exactly is it? Imagine energy as an unseen force whirling around the world, ready to be tapped. Although you can't physically hold it in your hands, you can see the sun's energy as light, feel it as warmth, and see evidence of it in the life around you. You can hear the invisible energy of thunder during a rainstorm. The stimulating effects of a nutritious diet can make you more aware of your strength and stamina.

Positive mental energy can be transmitted through a kind word or a thoughtful gesture. Healing energy is conveyed through laying on of hands, Reiki, touch therapy, massage, or simple human contact. Energy can come in the form of inspiration, prayer, meditation, and exercise, as well as from time spent alone, in nature, and with family and friends.

We need large amounts of energy in order to survive and thrive and deal with the demands of modern life; sadly, most of us don't have nearly enough of this precious resource. It's an elusive, mysterious force that courses through our beings. We know when we have it; we know when it's flagging.

I hope these tips will help guide you toward recapturing your zest for life, your happiness, your wholeness, and your physical stamina.

Blessing of Abundant Energy to You and Yours,

Stephanie Tourles

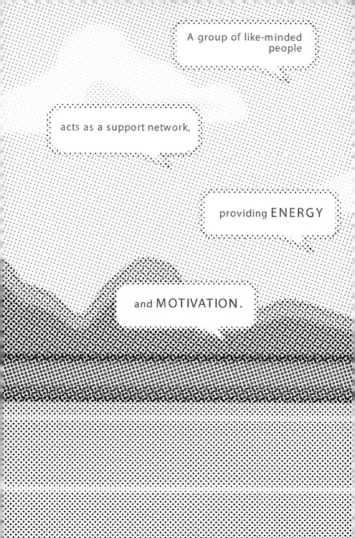

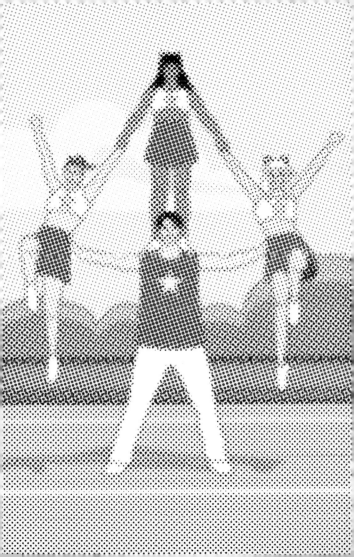

★
★

"IF YOU'VE EVER DONE ANYTHING
SUCCESSFULLY, YOU CAN DO IT
AGAIN. IMAGINE AND FEEL CERTAIN
NOW ABOUT THE EMOTIONS YOU
DESERVE TO HAVE INSTEAD OF
WAITING FOR THEM TO SPONTA-
NEOUSLY APPEAR SOMEDAY IN
THE FAR DISTANT FUTURE."

Anthony Robbins

"THE HUMAN SOUL NEEDS ACTUAL
BEAUTY MORE THAN BREAD."

D. H. Lawrence

A warm, luxuriant bath is the ultimate way to boost your circulation and balance your energy flow.

For a quick energy boost, place a few drops of peppermint, cypress, eucalyptus, spearmint, or geranium essential oil on a tissue and inhale deeply.

Drink eight glasses of water daily.

17

Believe in yourself and feel confident
that you can achieve anything you set
your mind to.

Follow your heart without asking
whether it's okay to do so.

"THIS IS THE TRUE JOY IN LIFE,
THE BEING USED FOR A PURPOSE
RECOGNIZED BY YOURSELF AS A
MIGHTY ONE."

George Bernard Shaw

Sleep is the best-kept beauty and energy secret around.

21

Visualize scenes of happiness, health, and success. Fill in the details with colors, sounds, and scents.

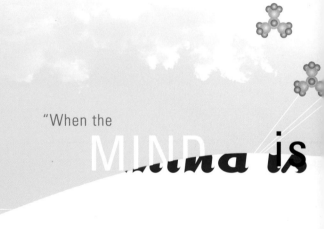

"When the **MIND** is

naginativelive .

it takes to itself the faintest hints of life, it converts
the very pulses of the air into revelations."

Henry James

"THE SHOE THAT FITS ONE
PERSON PINCHES ANOTHER;
THERE IS NO RECIPE FOR LIVING
THAT SUITS ALL CASES."

Carl Gustav Jung

25

Avoid the elevator; take the stairs instead.

Put an end to a bad relationship.

27

Mother Nature offers the best medicine for your soul.

Take some bread, crackers, or sunflower seeds to the park to spend some time with your feathered friends.

29

Update your look with a new haircut, makeup colors, or eyeglass frames.

"TAKE A MUSIC BATH ONCE OR TWICE
A WEEK FOR A FEW SEASONS AND
YOU WILL FIND THAT IT IS TO THE
SOUL WHAT THE WATER BATH IS TO
THE BODY."

Oliver Wendell Holmes

Studies reveal that the more social
connections you have, the better
your overall health.

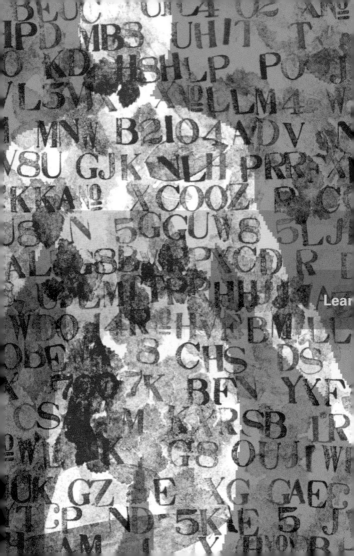

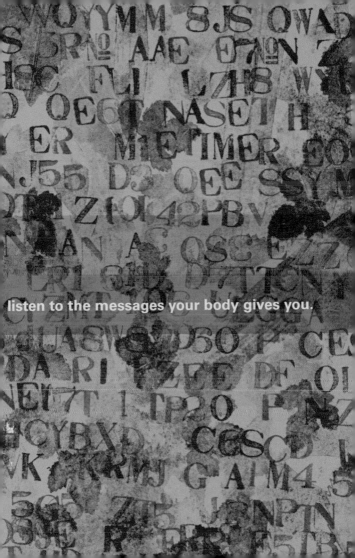

listen to the messages your body gives you.

Polarity therapy is a holistic approach to healing that gently manipulates your muscles to unblock energy flow and rebalance your body.

"THOSE WHO DARE AND DARE GREATLY
ARE THOSE WHO ACHIEVE."

Anonymous

Reiki is a Japanese healing therapy through which the practitioner channels the vital energy of the universe to remove energy blockages and revitalize your body.

Acupressure stimulates special points on the body to help relieve pain and boost energy without the use of acupuncture needles.

Treat your feet to a wooden footsie roller.

"THE PEOPLE WHO LIVE LONG
ARE THOSE WHO LONG TO LIVE."

Anonymous

Boredom can bring on chronic fatigue.

Exercise outside to help oxygenate your cells with fresh air and facilitate the removal of waste products through your skin.

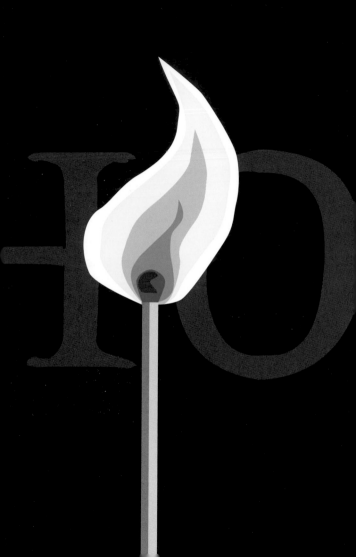

"Each time someone

stands up for an ideal,

or acts to improve the

lot of others, or strikes out

against injustice,

they send forth

a ripple of hope."

Robert F. Kennedy

Begin your day with some gentle
stretching exercises to get your
blood and oxygen flowing.

Ten to 15 minutes of unprotected exposure to sunlight several times a week is essential for healthy skin and bones.

Balance your energy by listening to recordings of nature sounds, such as a crashing surf, jungle rhythms, or bird songs.

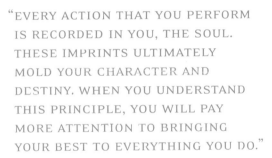

"EVERY ACTION THAT YOU PERFORM
IS RECORDED IN YOU, THE SOUL.
THESE IMPRINTS ULTIMATELY
MOLD YOUR CHARACTER AND
DESTINY. WHEN YOU UNDERSTAND
THIS PRINCIPLE, YOU WILL PAY
MORE ATTENTION TO BRINGING
YOUR BEST TO EVERYTHING YOU DO."

Dadi Janki

Studies show that pet owners live healthier, happier, less stressful lives.

49

Fresh, whole, unprocessed foods satisfy
your soul and nourish your body.

"I WAS ALWAYS LOOKING OUTSIDE
MYSELF FOR STRENGTH AND
CONFIDENCE BUT IT COMES FROM
WITHIN. IT IS THERE ALL THE TIME."

Anna Freud

51

Kick off your shoes and walk barefoot
in the grass.

make ¢

VISIT A LOCAL COSMETOLOGY
OR HAIRDRESSING SCHOOL

FOR A MAKEOVER AT A
FRACTION OF THE PRICE.

Rediscover the joys of an imaginative journey through reading.

55

Communicate with nature.

"THE STRONGEST PRINCIPLE OF
GROWTH LIES IN HUMAN CHOICE."

George Eliot

"A MAN BECOMES WHAT HE THINKS
ABOUT ALL DAY LONG."

Ralph Waldo Emerson

Eating several small meals rather than two or three large ones keeps your sugar level stable, prevents mood swings and headaches, and ensures a steady stream of nutrients throughout the day.

59

Letting go is an act of strength and courage. It helps healing begin, frees you of the weight of the past, and opens doors to a new future.

Touching another person exchanges healing energy, which results in a greater sense of well-being for both people.

61

Avoid coffee, black tea, soda, alcohol, and refined juices.

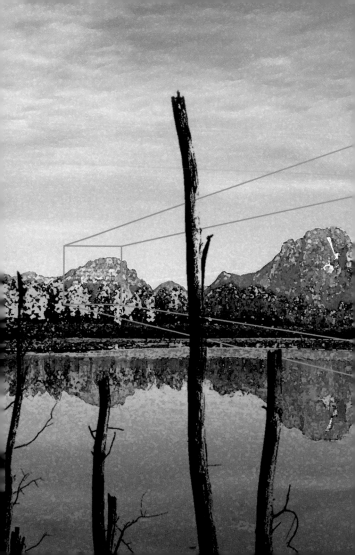

THE GOOD YOU DO TODAY
MAY BE QUICKLY FORGOTTEN,
BUT THE IMPACT OF WHAT YOU DO
WILL NEVER DISAPPEAR.

ANONYMOUS

Throw away your snow blower
and pick up a shovel.

Mow the lawn yourself.

Leave your car in the garage
and dust off that old bike.

Use your lunchtime to go outside,
breathe deeply, and move your body.

"WITHOUT THIS PLAYING WITH
FANTASY NO CREATIVE WORK HAS
EVER YET COME TO BIRTH."

Carl Gustav Jung

69

Look forward to something.

Wear red, orange, or yellow
to brighten your mood.

71

Be the kind of friend who laughs at all jokes, even if they're not that funny.

Swimming

makes you feel powerfu

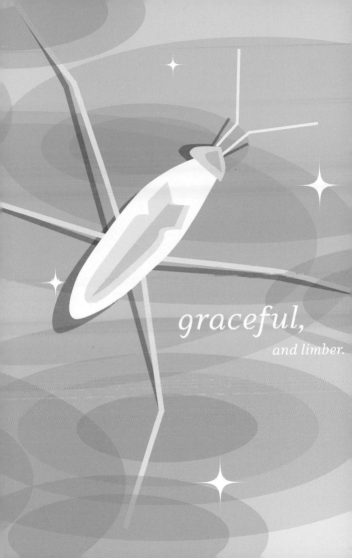

graceful,

and limber.

74

Train for a local fun run or benefit walk in your community.

75

"YOU JUST CAN'T BEAT THE PERSON
WHO NEVER GIVES UP."

George "Babe" Ruth

Splash cold water on your face and run your hands and wrists under the cold tap water.

"LIFE IS A DARING ADVENTURE
OR NOTHING."

Helen Keller

Learn to say "no" more often
to demanding friends, family,
and co-workers.

Clean up your emotional life by forgiving someone who has done you wrong.

Book a full-body massage.

Improve your posture: Walk around
your living room with a book balanced
on top of your head.

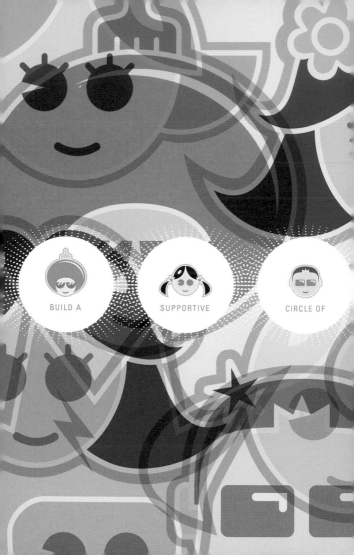

BUILD A   SUPPORTIVE   CIRCLE OF

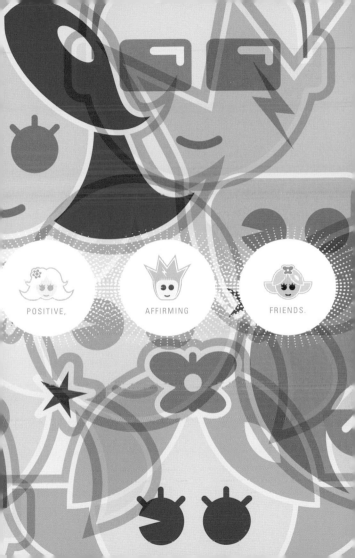

POSITIVE,

AFFIRMING

FRIENDS.

Raise your metabolic rate with spices such as cardamom, ginger, cinnamon, onions, chili pepper, black pepper, garlic, and hot mustard.

Chocolate increases the levels of mood-boosting hormones in your brain and is a source of the anti-depressant phenylethylamine.

Get rid of so-called "friends" who are negative or who bring you down.

Put a scented geranium near a sunny window and gently rub the leaves between your fingers when you need a lift.

Singing draws more oxygen into your body, enhances mental clarity, and banishes fatigue.

Laughter makes you feel good, makes your skin glow, and stimulates circulation and oxygen throughout your body.

"EVERY DAY IS A BIRTHDAY; EVERY MOMENT OF IT IS NEW TO US; WE ARE BORN AGAIN, RENEWED FOR FRESH WORK AND ENDEAVOR."

Issac Watts

Ginkgo Biloba boosts circulation to the brain, enhancing memory and alertness.

ENJOY THE

LITTLE

PLEASURES.

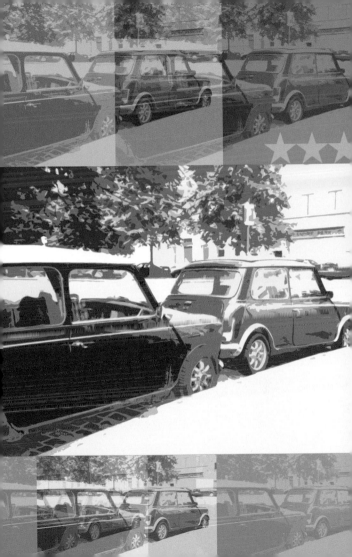

Keeping a journal is a soul-enriching experience.

Take a hike or a walk.

"CHEERFULNESS AND CONTENT
ARE GREAT BEAUTIFIERS AND
ARE FAMOUS PRESERVERS OF
YOUTHFUL LOOKS."

Charles Dickens

Research has shown that people who eat breakfast have higher metabolic rates than people who skip this vitally important meal.

Think about what makes you feel
attractive, strong, smart, or energetic.

"DEVELOP INTEREST IN LIFE AS YOU SEE IT; IN PEOPLE, THINGS, LITERATURE, MUSIC — THE WORLD IS SO RICH, SIMPLY THROBBING WITH RICH TREASURES, BEAUTIFUL SOULS AND INTERESTING PEOPLE."

Henry Miller

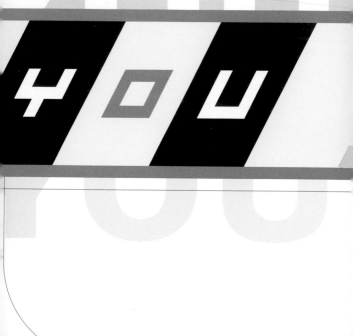

WHETHER YOU THINK YOU CAN, OR THINK

YOU

YOU

YOU

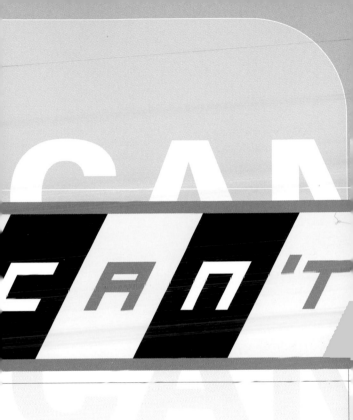

WHETHER YOU THINK YOU CAN OR YOU THINK YOU **CAN'T**.

YOU'RE PROBABLY RIGHT.

★ HENRY FORD ★

Value yourself as much as you expect others to value you.

"MOST OF US WILL MISS OUT ON
LIFE'S BIG PRIZES: THE PULITZERS,
THE HEISMANS, THE OSCARS. BUT
WE'RE ALL ELIGIBLE FOR A PAT ON
THE BACK, A KISS ON THE CHEEK, A
THUMBS-UP SIGN."

Barbara Johnson

Cultivate close friendships
and renew old ones.

Remember your past accomplishments.

Decide what you want for your future.

The act of being mindful opens you to the full experience of the moment.

Every big change begins with a baby step.

"AFFIRMATION OF LIFE IS THE SPIRITUAL ACT BY WHICH MAN CEASES TO LIVE UNREFLECTIVELY AND BEGINS TO DEVOTE HIMSELF TO HIS LIFE WITH REVERENCE IN ORDER TO RAISE IT TO ITS TRUE VALUE."

Albert Schweitzer

The man who has planted a garden feels that he has done something for the good of the whole world.

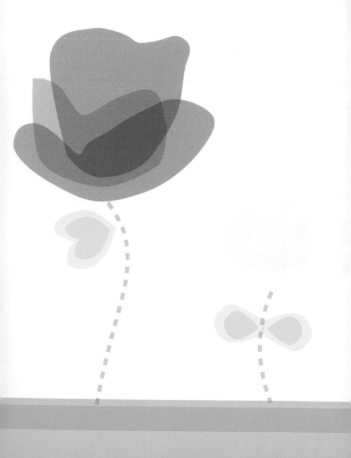

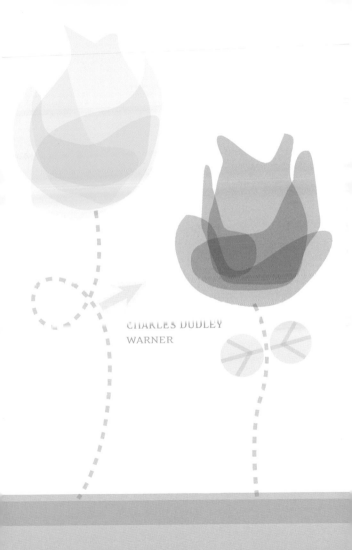

CHARLES DUDLEY
WARNER

What we manifest in this life is a reflection of what dwells deep inside us: If we want to renew our lives, we have to change our inner beliefs.

Stretch yourself beyond your usual limits.

Paint the walls of a room a vibrant color.

Take a long walk in the light
of the full moon.

"ONE WHO PLANTS A GARDEN,
PLANTS HAPPINESS."

Anonymous

"HAPPINESS LIES IN THE
FULFILLMENT OF THE SPIRIT
THROUGH THE BODY."

Cyril Connolly

"MANY PERSONS HAVE A WRONG IDEA
OF WHAT CONSTITUTES REAL HAPPI-
NESS. IT IS NOT OBTAINED THROUGH
SELF-GRATIFICATION BUT THROUGH
FIDELITY TO A WORTHY PURPOSE."

Helen Keller

Ask yourself with gentleness and patience, "In my heart of hearts, what do I really want?"

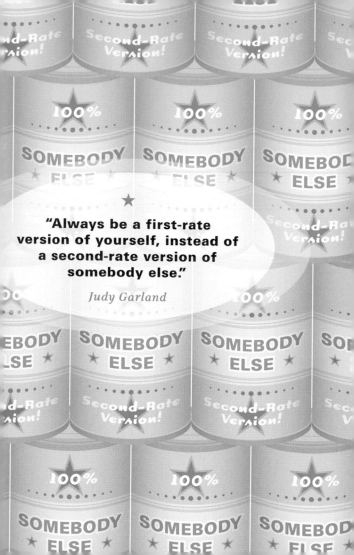

"Always be a first-rate version of yourself, instead of a second-rate version of somebody else."

Judy Garland

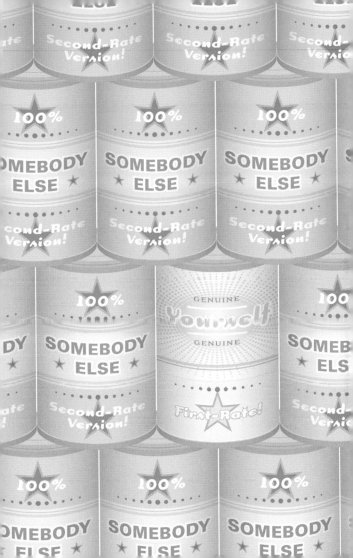

Pursue only those things in life that
support harmony, balance, inspiration,
and spiritual enlightenment.

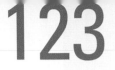

Allow your experiences — good and bad — to nourish your spirit and give you strength.

Reclaim your personal time and you'll naturally reclaim your own energy.

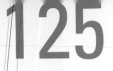

Known as the stone of nobility, the blood-red ruby is said to gather and amplify energy while promoting and stimulating mental concentration.

"INSTEAD OF MEASURING YOUR
LIFE'S VALUE BY YOUR PROGRESS
TOWARD A SINGLE GOAL, REMEMBER
THAT THE DIRECTION YOU'RE
HEADED IN IS MORE IMPORTANT
THAN TEMPORARY RESULTS."

Anthony Robbins

Read books, watch movies, attend plays, visit museums, take classes.

Vibrant shades of red have an
energy-boosting, highly stimulating
effect on the body.

"TRY A THING YOU HAVEN'T DONE
THREE TIMES. ONCE, TO GET OVER
THE FEAR OF DOING IT. TWICE, TO
LEARN HOW TO DO IT. AND A THIRD
TIME TO FIGURE OUT WHETHER YOU
LIKE IT OR NOT."

Virgil Thomson

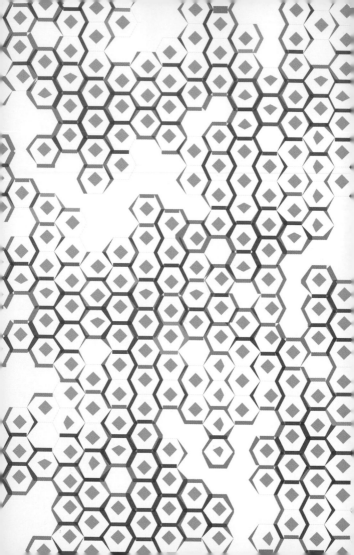

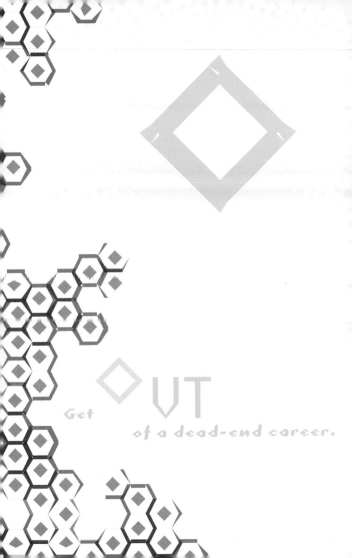

Get Out of a dead-end career.

"YOUR SOUL HAS DESIGNED THIS
LIFE FOR YOU IN ORDER FOR YOU TO
LEARN ITS LESSONS. BE GRATEFUL
FOR ALL THOSE PEOPLE WHO HAVE
BEEN YOUR TEACHERS."

Robin Norwood

Constant noise can be stressful
and physically exhausting.

See if you can still do a handstand,
a cartwheel, or a round-off.

The color orange relieves fatigue and depression and enhances creativity.

The color green balances your energy.

Violet, the color of royalty, stimulates self-confidence and joy.

"GIVE ME BEAUTY IN THE INWARD
SOUL; AND MAY THE INNER AND
OUTER BE AT ONE."

Plato

"SELF-REVERENCE, SELF-KNOWLEDGE,
SELF-CONTROL. THESE THREE ALONE
LEAD LIFE TO SOVEREIGN POWER."

Alfred, Lord Tennyson

DROP

★★ IF ON

FROM YOUR
VOCABULARY.

★ ★

"WORK IS LOVE MADE VISIBLE."

Kahlil Gibran

Zinc helps increase endurance
and prevents fatigue.

Shiatsu, a form of Japanese acupressure massage, is designed to establish balance within the body by applying pressure at strategic energy points on the body.

Known for its ability to promote longevity and increase endurance, bee pollen is available in granular form from health food stores.

Did you know that staying physically fit as you age also helps maintain mental fitness?

"WHAT WOULD YOU ATTEMPT TO DO IF
YOU KNEW YOU COULD NOT FAIL?"

Anonymous

Hang a squirrel-proof bird feeder in front of a sunny window that you frequently pass during the day.

"THE LOVE FOR ALL LIVING
CREATURES IS THE MOST
NOBLE ATTRIBUTE."

Charles Darwin

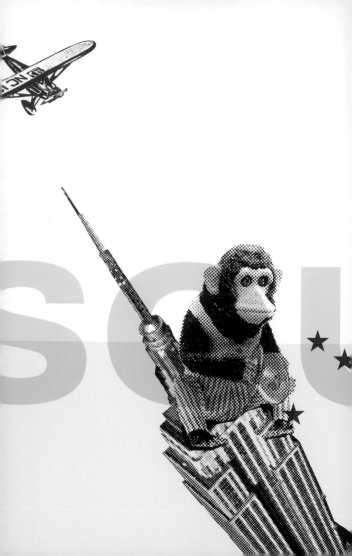

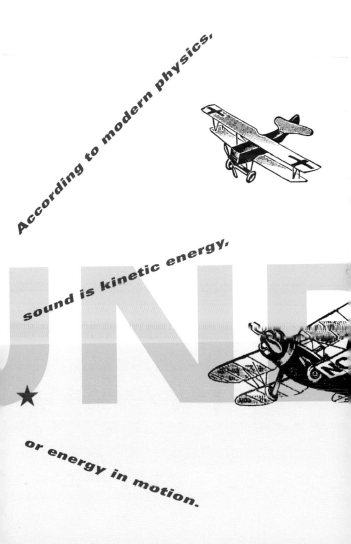

According to modern physics,

sound is kinetic energy,

or energy in motion.

Creating and cooking a great meal
can recharge your mind and body.

153

Lifting weights enhances
your metabolism.

Believe it or not, housework burns about 250 calories per hour, energizing your body.

Learn to love your body in all its strengths and weaknesses.

"EVEN IF IT'S A LITTLE THING,
DO SOMETHING FOR WHICH
YOU GET NO PAY BUT THE
PRIVILEGE OF DOING IT."

Albert Schweitzer

Seek out the beauty in your locale and revel in it as often as possible.

"FAITH IS IN MANY WAYS LIKE A
WHEELBARROW. YOU HAVE TO PUT
SOME REAL PUSH BEHIND IT TO
MAKE IT WORK."

Anonymous

Smoking can cause fatigue because it depletes the amount of oxygen in your bloodstream.

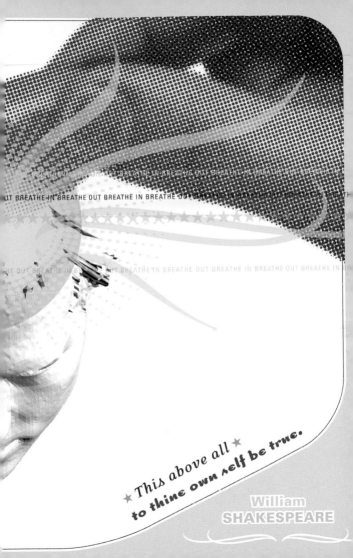

BREATHE IN BREATHE OUT BREATHE IN BREATHE OUT BREATHE IN BREATHE OUT BREATHE IN BREATHE OUT BREATHE IN BREATHE OUT

OUT BREATHE IN BREATHE OUT BREATHE IN BREATHE OUT BREATHE IN BREATHE OUT BREATHE IN BREATHE OUT BREATHE IN BREATH

HE OUT BREATHE IN BREATHE OUT BREATHE IN BREATHE OUT BREATHE IN BREATHE OUT BREATHE IN BREATHE OUT BREATHE IN BR

This above all ★
to thine own self be true.

William
SHAKESPEARE

The blue-green turquoise stone is believed to protect the wearer from negative energy.

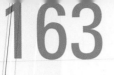

To achieve a larger goal,
start by implementing small,
easily manageable steps.

"INSIDE MYSELF IS A PLACE WHERE I
LIVE ALL ALONE AND THAT'S WHERE
YOU RENEW YOUR SPRINGS THAT
NEVER DRY UP."

Pearl S. Buck

Reliving fun memories will give you a lift

A quick spritz of cool water on your face will instantly revive your flagging energy and hydrate your skin.

Open the curtains, lift the shades, add a few lamps with full-spectrum light bulbs, and let the sun shine in.

Drink a large glass of ice-cold water or tea to shock your system into alertness.

"THERE IS SOMETHING INFINITELY
HEALING IN THE REPEATED REFRAINS
OF NATURE — THE ASSURANCE THAT
DAWN COMES AFTER NIGHT, AND
SPRING AFTER THE WINTER."

Rachel Carson

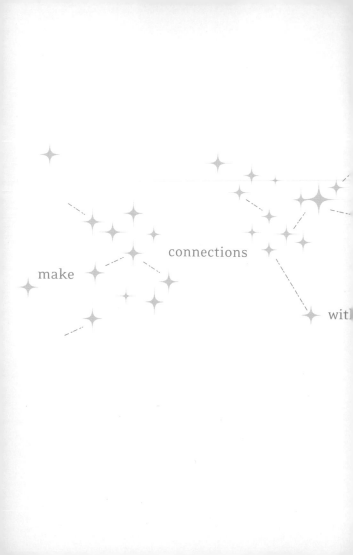

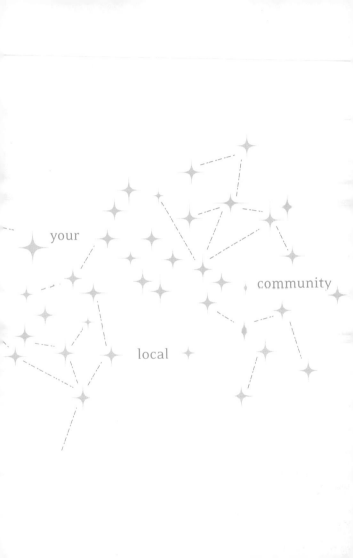

your

community

local

"THE SOUL SHOULD ALWAYS STAND
AJAR, READY TO WELCOME THE
ECSTATIC EXPERIENCE."

Emily Dickinson

High-fat meals divert blood away from your muscles, brain, and tissues.

The mind and heart need continued emotional and spiritual growth and a fulfillment of dreams, goals, and desires. These are the foods on which our souls thrive.

"TO LOVE ONESELF IS THE BEGINNING
OF A LIFELONG ROMANCE."

Oscar Wilde

A table adorned in bright, cheery colors will lift your mood every time you sit down for a meal.

Redecorate part of your house
or apartment.

Place a few drops of neroli essential oil on a handkerchief and deeply inhale — the fragrance balances and uplifts the psyche.

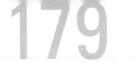

★
★

"WHEN I GO INTO MY GARDEN WITH A
SPADE, AND DIG A BED, I FEEL SUCH
AN EXHILARATION AND HEALTH
THAT I DISCOVER THAT I HAVE BEEN
DEFRAUDING MYSELF ALL THIS TIME
IN LETTING OTHERS DO FOR ME
WHAT I SHOULD HAVE DONE WITH
MY OWN HANDS."

Ralph Waldo Emerson

"Live each season
as it passes

DRINK THE DRINK, BREATHE THE AIR.

HENRY
DAVID
THOREAU

taste the fruit,
and resign
yourself to the
influences of each. **"**

If you eat until you're stuffed and don't listen to your body's signals of fullness, your energy will wane.

Add fuel to your furnace
by consuming more pumpkin.

Take a music appreciation course.

Watch the sunrise and absorb the oranges, yellows, pinks, and reds into your innermost being.

"...CREATIVITY ALWAYS MEANS THE DOING OF THE UNFAMILIAR, THE BREAKING OF NEW GROUND..."

Eleanor Roosevelt

Unclutter and organize your work area
so you won't be distracted by the mess
or by another project.

"SOUL DOESN'T POUR INTO LIFE
AUTOMATICALLY. IT REQUIRES
OUR SKILL AND ATTENTION."

Thomas Moore

According to Traditional Chinese Medicine, qi, or life energy, is expressed in vastly different forms through animals, humans, minerals, and plants, yet it unifies the physical, mental, and spiritual qualities of energy throughout the universe.

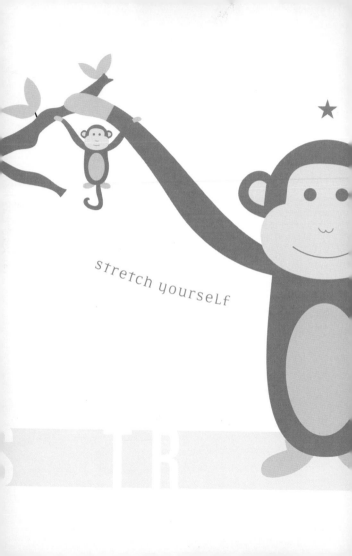

stretch yourself

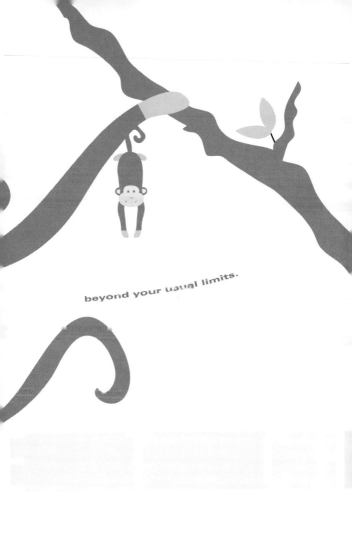

beyond your usual limits.

The amethyst is believed to transmit stability, invigoration, and strength.

Goldenrod flower essence repels
negativity and promotes positive
actions and thoughts.

"THERE CAN BE NO JOY OF LIFE
WITHOUT JOY OF WORK."

Thomas Aquinas

Considered the stone of health, the garnet is believed to extract negative energy from the body's chakras, creating a more balanced state.

Penstemon flower essence
promotes inner fortitude.

"THE MOST BEAUTIFUL THING
WE CAN EXPERIENCE IS THE
MYSTERIOUS. IT IS THE SOURCE
OF ALL TRUE ART AND SCIENCE."

Albert Einstein

Volunteer. You'll get a spiritual boost by helping others and the realization that your current circumstances aren't so bad after all.

Intentionally making an effort to change your physiology will produce an uplifted emotional state.

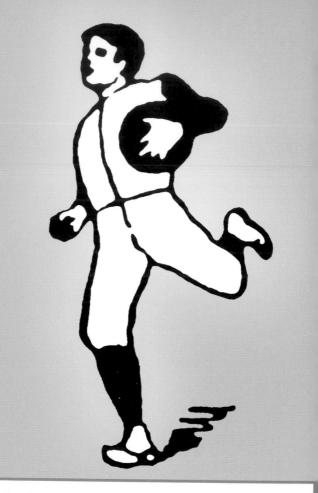

Exercise outside to help oxygenate your cells with fresh air

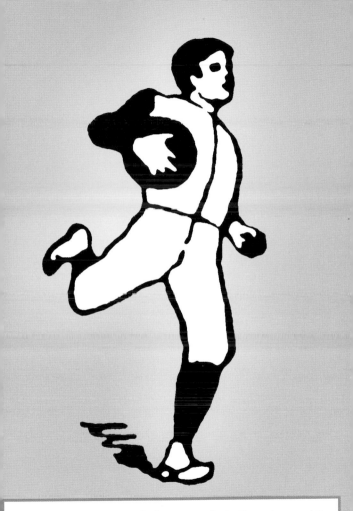

and facilitate the removal of waste products through your skin.

The rhodochrosite stone is believed to enhance spirituality and stimulate the vital energy of the body for optimal health.

"THERE IS A SINGLE MAGIC,
A SINGLE POWER,
A SINGLE SALVATION,
AND A SINGLE HAPPINESS,
AND THAT IS CALLED LOVING."

Herman Hesse

Increase the circulation of qi, or life energy, throughout your body and mind through yoga, dance, sports, moderate aerobic exercise, the martial arts, playing, and laughing.

Share in someone else's joyous moment and the happiness will become contagious.

Copper stimulates metabolism
and is believed to bring good luck
to those in its presence.

Next time raspberries, blackberries, strawberries, blueberries, or huckleberries are in season, visit a local berry farm or a friend with a backyard patch and pick a pail full of berries.

"WHATEVER YOU BELIEVE YOU CAN
DO OR DREAM YOU CAN, BEGIN IT.
BOLDNESS HAS GENIUS, POWER,
AND MAGIC IN IT."

Anonymous

Create a spiritual path through
daily meditation or prayer.

spread love

everywhere you go;

first of all in your own house.

Mother Teresa

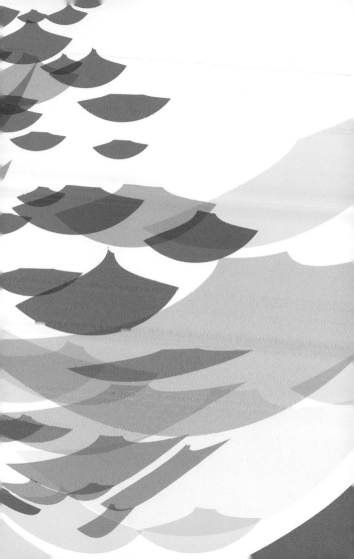

Art has no rules; it is not black or white, right or wrong.

"ENJOY LIFE'S 'PUDDLES.' MAKE
CHEERFULNESS, OUTRAGEOUSNESS,
AND PLAYFULNESS NEW PRIORITIES
FOR YOUR LIFE. YOU CAN FEEL GOOD
FOR NO REASON AT ALL!"

Anthony Robbins

"HOPE, ENTHUSIASM, AND
WISDOM ARE TO THE MIND
AS FOOD IS TO THE BODY."

Dadi Janki

The type of sound created by a large choir or your city's symphony orchestra can affect your body and mind in profound, positive ways, creating balance, well-being, and motivation.

Read the biography of someone you admire for inspiration.

"SHOOT FOR THE MOON. EVEN
IF YOU MISS IT YOU WILL LAND
AMONG THE STARS."

Les Brown

The yellow sapphire, yellow topaz, amber, and citrine stones are believed to increase energy and vitality.

"A FRIEND IS A PERSON WITH WHOM I MAY BE SINCERE. BEFORE HIM, I MAY THINK ALOUD."

Ralph Waldo Emerson

we never know

how high we are

till we are asked to rise;

and then, if we are true to plan,

our statures touch the skies.   EMILY DICKINSON

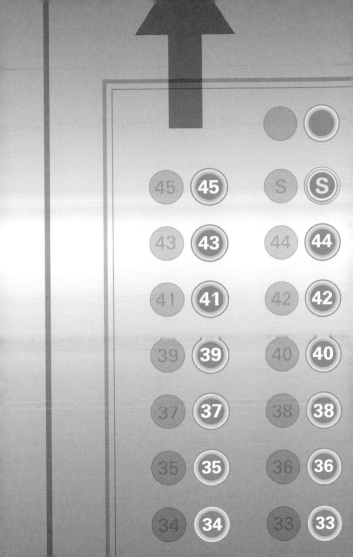

Worrying is unproductive and
fills your mind with unnecessary,
time-consuming thoughts.

"EACH MOMENT AND WHATEVER
HAPPENS THRILLS ME WITH JOY..."

Walt Whitman

Ask a loved one to give you a hug, hold your hand, brush your hair, rub your feet, or massage your shoulders. Then return the favor.

A mantra can consist of a single syllable, a string of syllables, a word, or a phrase and can be repeated aloud or silently to balance the body and mind.

"HAPPINESS IS NOT A DESTINATION. IT IS THE ATTITUDE WITH WHICH YOU CHOOSE TO TRAVEL."

Arit Desal

High in natural sugar, ripe bananas are storehouses of quick, healthy energy.

Manage your money!

In-line skating is a fun exercise for the whole family.

Don't wait for "the right moment"
to start a new project — that moment
may never come.

Be the kind of friend who is supportive
no matter what the circumstances.

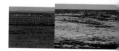

"Think of the fierce energy
concentrated in an acorn!

━►

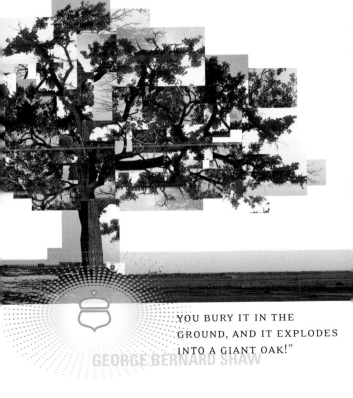

"YOU BURY IT IN THE
GROUND, AND IT EXPLODES
INTO A GIANT OAK!"

GEORGE BERNARD SHAW

"WE SHOULD CONSIDER EVERY DAY
LOST IN WHICH WE HAVE NOT
DANCED AT LEAST ONCE."

Fredrick Nietzsche

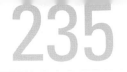

"THE MOON HAS PHASES FROM DARK
TO FULL. SO DO WE."

Victoria Moran

Learn a new creative pursuit, such as quilting, gardening, cooking new types of food, or anything that will bring you lasting delight.

Take a walk outdoors after a
thunder and lightning storm.

"FALLING IN LOVE AT FIRST SIGHT IS AS FINAL AS IT IS SWIFT...BUT THE GROWTH OF TRUE FRIENDSHIP MAY BE A LIFELONG AFFAIR."

Sarah Orne Jewett

Awaken a sluggish digestive system
by eating dandelion leaves.

Try to help someone every day.

One of the basic causes of illness is unhappiness, and one of the greatest healers is joy.

Wake up and decide that today
will be extraordinary!

Hug someone every day.

CALM ME DOWN

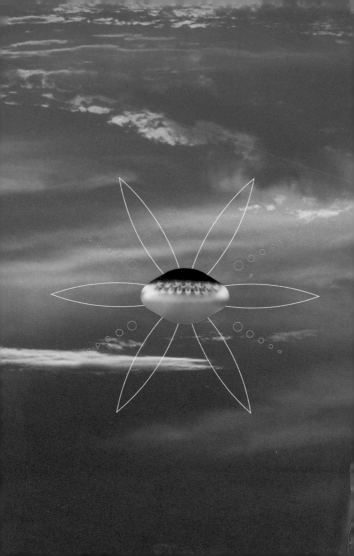

CALM ME DOWN

RELAX, SOOTHE, AND NURTURE YOUR BODY & MIND

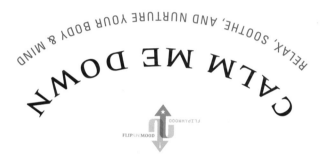

Barbara L. Heller

The mission of Storey Publishing is to serve our customers by publishing practical information that encourages personal independence in harmony with the environment.

Edited by Deborah Balmuth and Carey L. Boucher
Art direction by Joshua C. Chen and Cindy McFarland
Book design and illustrations by Chen Design Associates

Printed in Hong Kong by Elegance
10 9 8 7 6 5 4 3 2 1

Library of Congress Cataloging-in-Publication Data

Tourles, Stephanie.
    Lift me up, calm me down / by Stephanie Tourles and Barbara L. Heller.
        p. cm.
    ISBN 1-58017-163-X (alk. paper)
    1. Health. 2. Vitality. 3. Stress management. I. Tourles, Stephanie L. 1962- II. Title.

RA776.H484 2003
613—dc21   2003050559

To my husband, Alan

Acknowledgments

Heartfelt appreciation to my wonderful circle of support, most notably those who were in on the original project that grew into this book: Phyllis Heller, Paula Kephart, Suzanne Massa, Zach Rosen, Barbara Ruchames, Bob Ruchames, Tess Taft, and Irene Zahava.

A special thanks to Deborah Balmuth and the other great folks at Storey for the opportunities, guidance, and support.

My gratitude to my fantastic family: Alan and Rebecca, you continue to be my primary sources for inspiration, connection, wonder, and love.

REMEMBER TO RELAX

Are you feeling stressed? If so, you are not alone. The pace and pressures of modern life — our personal expectations as well as outside demands — are exhausting.

Most of us have not been taught to relax. But relaxation is an acquired skill — one that you can learn. True relaxation creates a calm center where you can return after stressful events. It also provides a peaceful counterpoint to positive stimulation. Releasing tension improves your immunity and heightens your creativity, effectiveness, intuition, and joy.

The most effective relaxation techniques require some planning and aim to create long-term solutions to stress. I hope that you make time to take a yoga class, write in a journal, be outdoors, connect with others, learn new

remedies, and experience serenity in silence. All take time and commitment.

But we also need small gems in our daily lives to help us practice. Use the simple suggestions here to augment your larger stress-management repertoire. When you can't get away from it all, when you are in the midst of the tension tornado, just stop for a second: Take a deep breath, page through this book, and reflect. The first step in stopping the stress cycle is to change your perspective. This step can be short, sweet, and immediate.

Please try some of the soul soothers in this book to help you to become more mellow and mindful. These stress-management soundbytes can become your best *reminders to relax*.

Barbara L. Heller, MSW

TURN **off** THE TELEVISION

Treat yourself to a sensual eye pillow.

Ask for help.

13

"FINISH EACH DAY AND BE DONE WITH IT. YOU HAVE DONE WHAT YOU COULD. TOMORROW IS A NEW DAY; BEGIN IT WELL AND SERENELY AND WITH TOO HIGH A SPIRIT TO BE ENCUMBERED WITH YOUR OLD NONSENSE."

Ralph Waldo Emerson

14

Carry a favorite magazine or paperback book in your bag to while away the time spent in waiting rooms and supermarket lines pleasantly.

15

If you break the fatigue-inactivity cycle with a jog or an aerobics class, you will be rewarded with relaxation.

16

Relax with the sedating scents of lavender, lemon balm, Roman chamomile, neroli, ylang ylang, and clary sage.

Figure out the reasons for your procrastination, then don't delay!

18

Write your own horoscope.
Live today with that possibility.

19

"May you have warm
words on a cold evening,
a full moon on a dark night,

and the road

DOWNHILL

all the way to your door."

Mary Engelbreit

Schedule a worry session. If you honor your concerns for a focused half-hour, you may eliminate being plagued by worries throughout the day.

22

Write a list of relaxing words
on an index card and keep it
at your desk as a reminder.

"IF YOU TAKE YOUR TIME AND KEEP YOUR WITS ABOUT YOU, YOU CAN CULTIVATE A WHOLESOME AND ARTFUL SPIRITUAL LIFE THAT NOURISHES THE WHOLE SELF — ONE THAT WILL HELP YOU ENJOY THE WORLD AND PERHAPS EVEN SAVE IT."

Elizabeth Lesser

24

Letting go of an old regret or shameful memory is often difficult but always liberating.

25

Valerian is the premier herb to
treat insomnia and stress.

Don't be embarrassed — reading sappy, silly, or simple books is a wonderful form of no-stress entertainment.

27

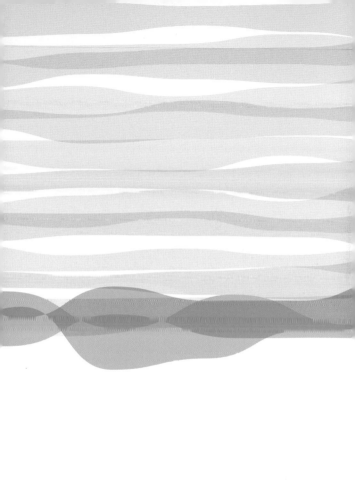

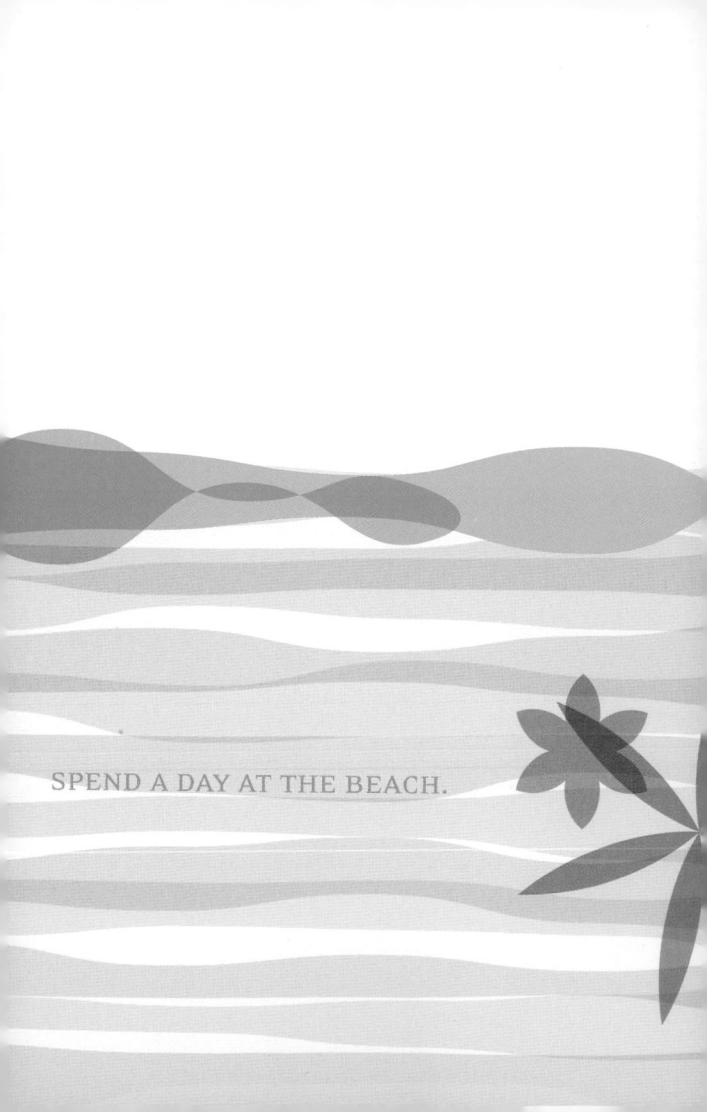

SPEND A DAY AT THE BEACH.

30

Relive pleasant memories.

"MOVING TOWARD AN INWARDLY SIMPLE LIFE IS NOT ABOUT DEPRIVATION OR DENYING OURSELVES THE THINGS WE WANT. IT'S ABOUT GETTING RID OF THE THINGS THAT NO LONGER CONTRIBUTE TO THE FULLNESS OF OUR LIVES. IT'S ABOUT CREATING BALANCE BETWEEN OUR INNER AND OUTER LIVES."

Elaine St. James

31

Enhance the spiritual meaning of the holiday season while eliminating credit card debt — limit gifts to a preplanned amount.

Where can you go to renew your
connection with nature?

Choose a comforting
commuting companion.

34

Go fly a kite.

35

Choose a versatile wash-and-wear hair style that looks attractive and lessens morning primp time.

Humor is healing.

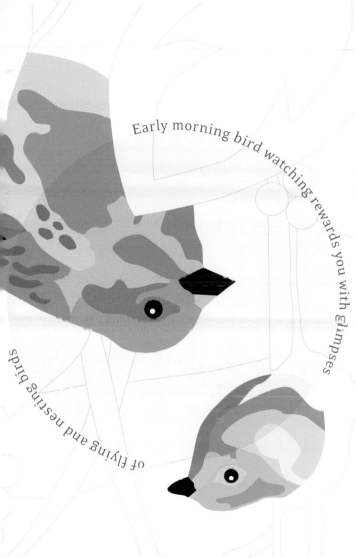

Early morning bird watching rewards you with glimpses of flying and nesting birds

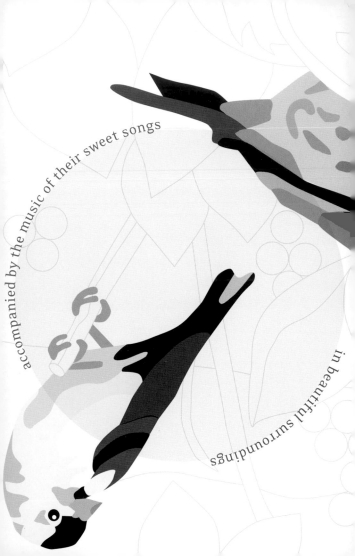

accompanied by the music of their sweet songs

in beautiful surroundings

41

During rush hour, calm down
by listening to Sylvia Boorstein's
Road Sage on audio cassette.

40

Live with a poem for a week.

42

Walk barefoot.

Plan a personal pampering party.

Catnip, a tasty and easy-to-grow cousin
of mint, makes a mild sedative tea.

Surround yourself with items that don't demand a lot of extra care.

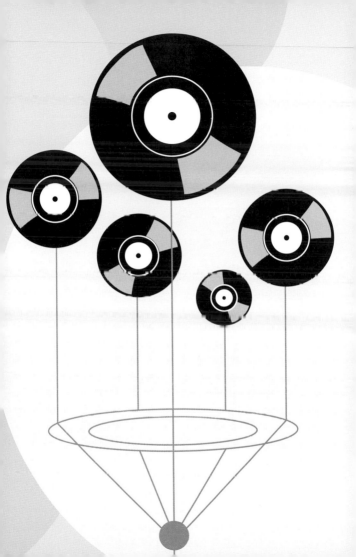

soothing sound to the ear than CDs and. Records provide a more

Pencil in your planner a personal deadline that is days or weeks before the actual deadline.

48

Simmer a small amount of cloves, cinnamon, and orange peel in two cups of water on top of the stove. The soothing fragrance will fill your home.

"BEAUTY OF STYLE AND HARMONY AND GRACE
AND GOOD RHYTHM DEPEND ON SIMPLICITY."

Plato

50

Cleaning out your closets lessens the amount you have to organize, clean, and repair. And that frees up time to relax.

Attend a monthly meditation meeting.

52

Pour yourself a tall, chilled glass
of chamomile or lemon balm tea and
garnish with a sprig of fresh mint.

54

Don't bring work home.

Serve yourself a glass of ice-cold lemonade and sip it through a straw.

"*You must* learn to be still in the midst of ac*tivity*

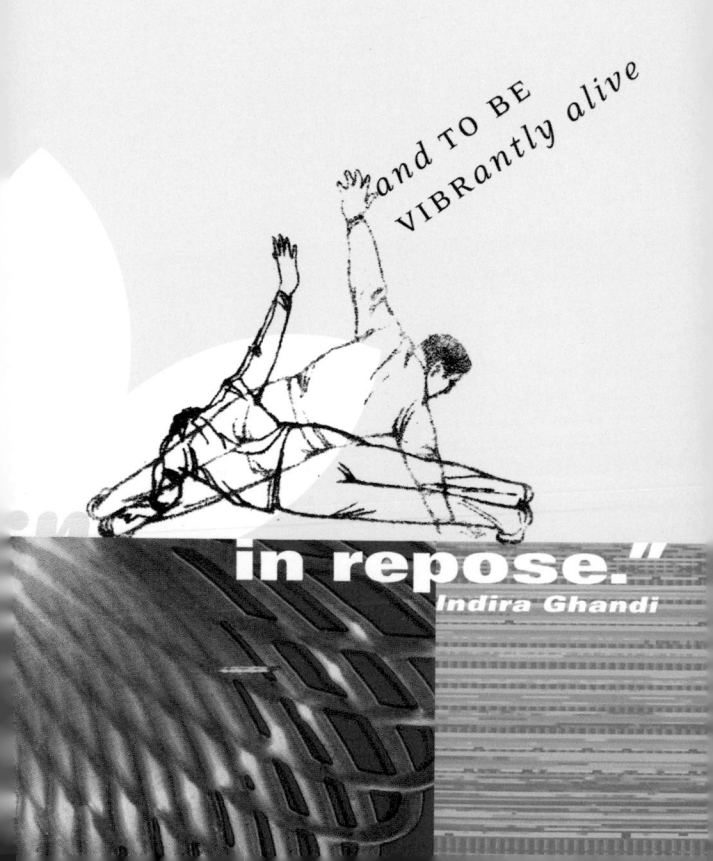

"...and TO BE VIBRantly alive VIBRantly alive in repose."

—Indira Ghandi

Invite your family or friends to a
movie marathon – at home.

58

Just say "no" to requests for
your participation.

Allow extra time for your morning drive.

60

Eat on the porch or picnic in the park.

Turn off the alarm clock.

"THERE WILL BE ENOUGH TIME TO DO IT ALL.
BUT NOT ALL AT ONCE."

Wayne Sotile

63

64

Explore a place of enchantment.

Treat yourself to some refined relaxation. Ask a friend to accompany you to a play, art film, ballet, or opera.

65

TRAVEL DOWN THE HIGHWAY
WITHOUT A DESTINATION.

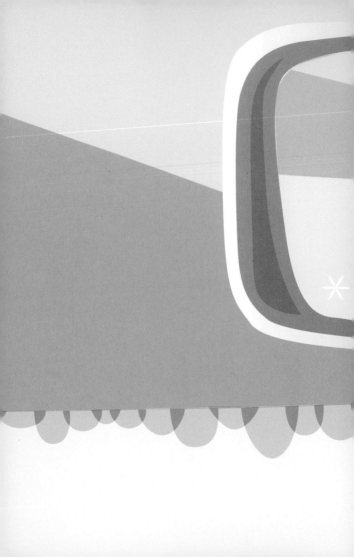

"BE WILLING TO LIVE IN BETWEEN RIGHT AND WRONG. THE EGO NEEDS AND DESPERATELY WANTS TO BE RIGHT AND MAKE OTHERS WRONG. IN BETWEEN RIGHT AND WRONG IS A SOFT, MESSY, LAUGHING PLACE WHERE IT DOESN'T MATTER."

Sark

68

Free up your free time for some really relaxing activities.

Vanilla's deep, sweet scent summons
a sense of calm.

Choose a theme for holiday gifts, such as books or kitchen supplies, and buy similar presents for everyone on your list.

The average adult needs seven to nine hours of sleep a night to function well.

Take a slow shower.

Indulge in comfortable bedding.

Tame your restless "monkey mind" with a mantra, a syllable or word silently repeated or softly spoken during meditation.

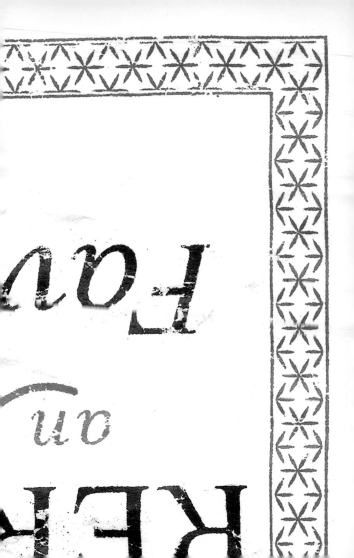

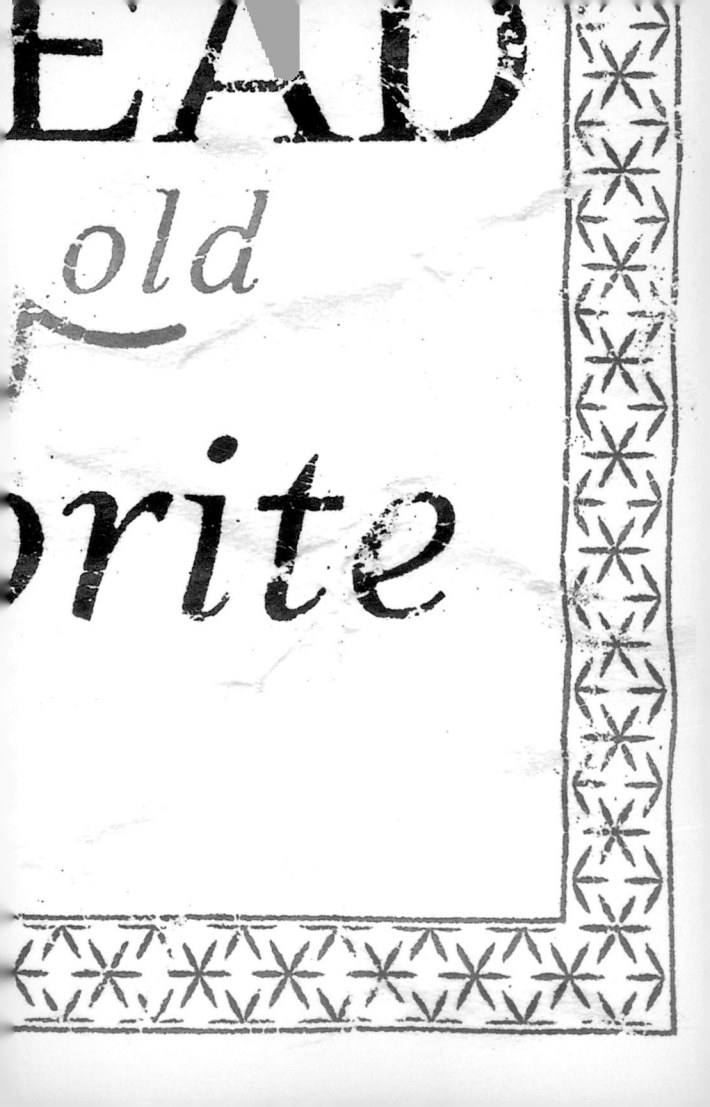

A sleep survey found that those who walked at least six blocks a day at a normal pace were one-third less likely to have trouble sleeping than nonwalkers.

Avoid alcoholic beverages before bedtime.

79

08

Design a bedtime ritual.

If you have problems sleeping, reset
your body clock by keeping to a curfew.

Spend time reading about a new-to-you field, such as science, historical fiction, relationships, or crafts.

82

Eat calming carbohydrates, such as bread, cereal, and pasta, to trigger the brain chemicals that make you sleepy.

Convert a cozy corner or empty room into a place to meditate.

84

"WE EMBARK UPON THE CREATION OF A
PEACEFUL LIFESTYLE BY RECOGNIZING
THE NEED, DAILY, TO CLEANSE OUR MINDS
JUST AS WE CLEANSE OUR BODIES.
THROUGH MORNING PRAYERS AND
MEDITATION, WE EMBARK UPON THE DAY
SPIRITUALLY PREPARED. WITHOUT THIS
PREPARATION, WE ENTER THE DAY WITH
YESTERDAY'S ANXIETIES — OUR OWN
AND THOSE OF MILLIONS OF OTHERS."

Marianne Williamson

85

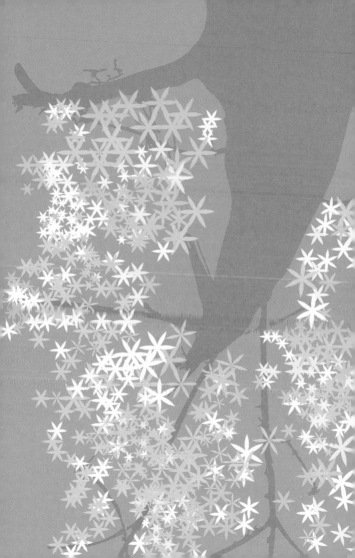

PLAYING IN A PILE OF AUTUMN LEAVES
is one of the best natural tranquilizers.

View only gentle beauty from your bed.

88

Do one thing at a time.

When you come home, change into comfortable, casual clothes, and leave your work concerns behind.

Take the day off.

Laughing reduces stress hormone levels, decreases blood pressure, and relieves muscle tension.

Appreciate the art of lazy days.

"THERE IS NOTHING WORTH MORE
THAN THIS DAY."

Johann Wolfgang von Goethe

94

Drink eight glasses of water every day.

Become aware of your posture.

Yawning relieves tension, fatigue,
and boredom.

Delight in the dawning of a new day.

A walk in the woods will improve your mood, provide you with a cardiovascular boost, and satisfy you visually.

100

"MY SPECIAL PLACE IS A SMALL BROOK
IN A GREEN GLADE, A CIRCLE OF QUIET
FROM WHICH THERE IS NO VISIBLE SIGN
OF HUMAN BEINGS. IF I SIT FOR A WHILE,
THEN MY IMPATIENCE, CROSSNESS,
FRUSTRATION ARE INDEED ANNIHILATED,
AND MY SENSE OF HUMOR RETURNS."

Madeleine L'Engle

101

Appreciate your own achievements.

Listen closely: The signs of serenity are often more subtle than the symptoms of stress.

104

Perfectionism produces anxiety.

Hang out in a hammock.

allow dinner
sturbed by
calls.

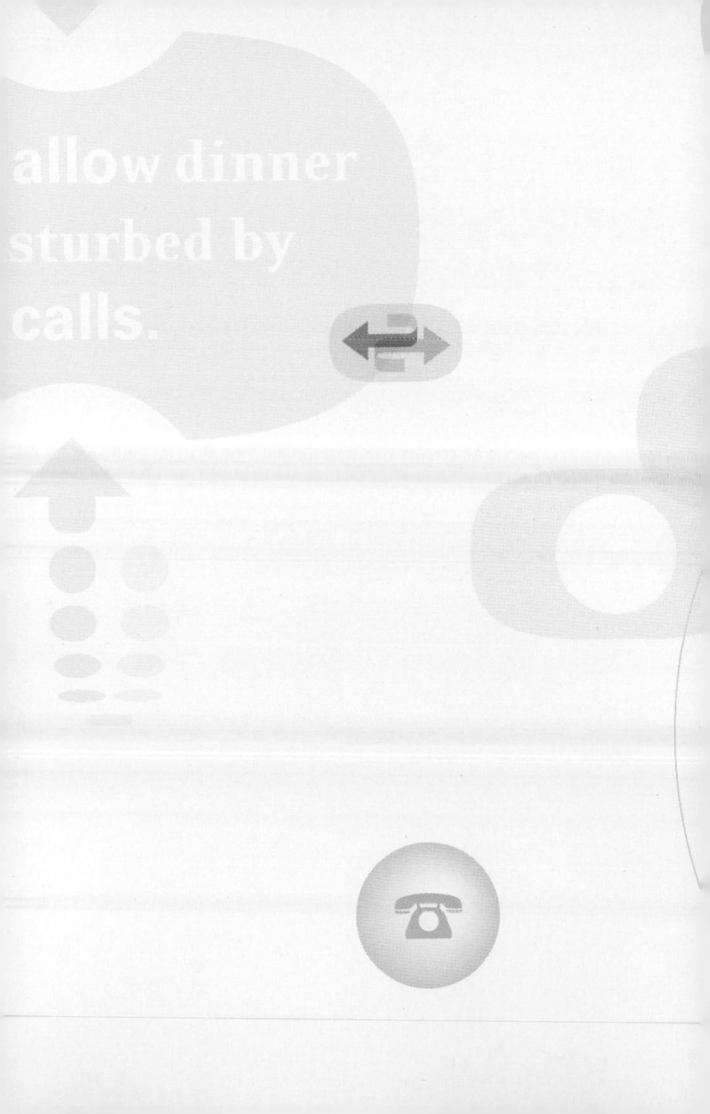

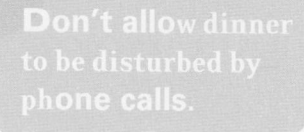

Don't allow dinner
to be disturbed by
phone calls.

108

Make peace with your past.

Find your dream job.

"TOMORROW IS NOT PROMISED, NOR IS TODAY.
SO I CHOOSE TO CELEBRATE EVERY DAY I'M
ALIVE BY BEING PRESENT IN IT. LIVING IN
THE PRESENT MEANS LETTING GO OF THE
PAST AND NOT WAITING FOR THE FUTURE."

Oprah Winfrey

110

Studies show that listening to calm instrumental music before bed will help you nod off more quickly.

Take a walk in the light of the moon.

Before a stressful or difficult event,
imagine yourself doing the task well.

Hang some wind chimes by your window, door, or porch, and listen to the soft music in the breeze.

People who regularly write about their stressful experiences have fewer symptoms of chronic illness and develop a greater sense of well-being.

115

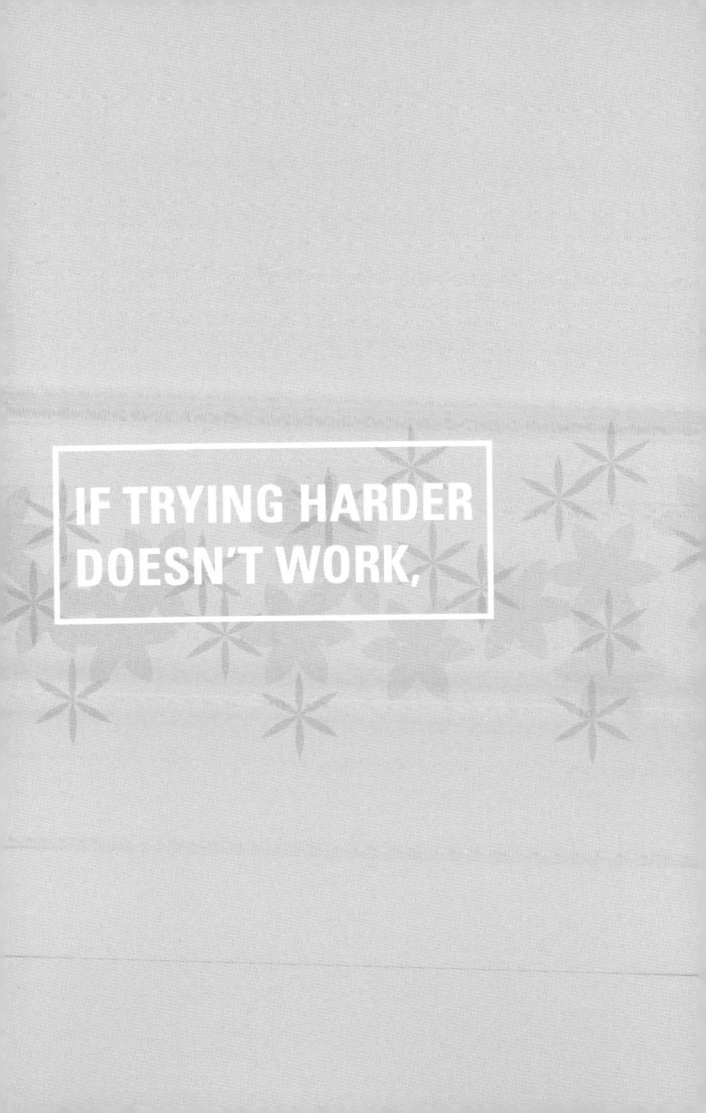

IF TRYING HARDER
DOESN'T WORK,

try softer.

Lily Tomlin

Notice the magical quality of dusk,
the time of in-between.

Share your space with other living things. Healthy potted plants and fish-filled aquariums create a calming effect in your home.

Using the language of imagery reduces stress, helps us resolve personal conflicts, and gives voice to our inner messages. Color your thoughts and emotions in shapes and images.

120

Savor a stunning sunset.

Listen to the sound of water —
the rhythm of ocean waves,
trickling waterfalls, rushing streams,
raindrops, or an indoor fountain.

Nourish your relationship with
your inner self by keeping a journal.

Turn off negative thoughts.

Pin up peaceful postcards to transform the mood of your workspace.

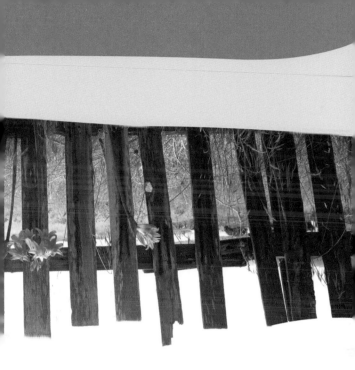

Simple pleasures are the best.

BOBBY MCFERRIN

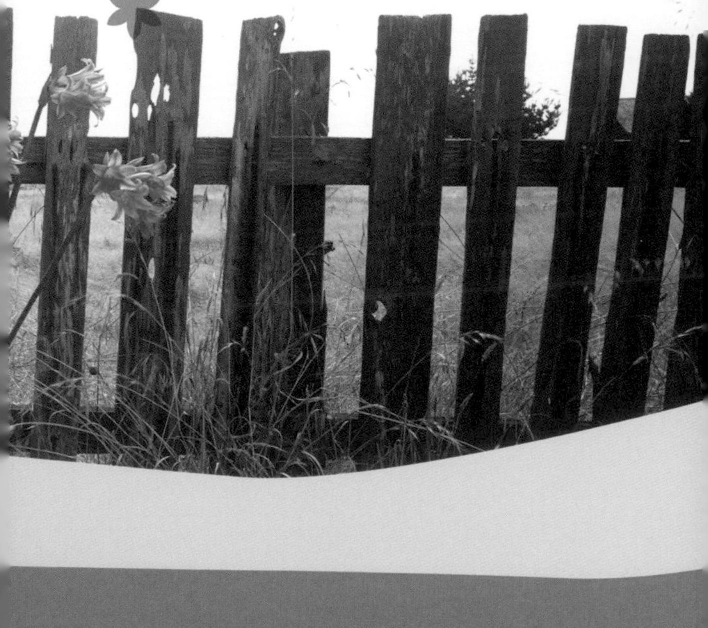

Find the perfect comfortable chair.

Lie down on the grass.

Set a tone of calm and comfort in the threshold to your home.

Warm feet are a natural sedative.

Remember that perspective is a habit.

Bake a batch of your favorite cookies.

The gardener's secret is that what appears to be hard work is also a salve for the soul.

People who write down their goals
are more successful in realizing them
than those who don't.

The winds of grace are

and it's up to us
to raise our sails

Father Thomas Keating

blowing

aLL the time,

Take a needed midday break.

Take time to smell the roses, literally.

There are two ways to positively deal with stress. You can change the stressful situation or change your physical and emotional responses to the stressful situation. Understanding your options is the first step to relaxation.

"HOW BEAUTIFUL IT IS TO DO NOTHING
AND REST AFTERWARDS."

Spanish proverb

Share in communal song – join a
choir, chant with a group, or conduct
a sing-along.

Experiment with simple ways to express yourself.

Seeing someone smile warms the heart
and lifts the spirit.

Pleasant recollections instill calm.

Bright natural light
early in the day

enhances your body's
internal rhythms

and helps you sleep
better at night.

Pull some weeds and trim some shrubs.
Both you and your yard will benefit.

Giving voice to your inner thoughts lets your heart and soul catch your attention.

Open the window and let the outdoors in.

150

Young children live only in the present moment. See the world from a child's point of view.

Throw something away.

Light incense to bring calm
to your space.

Loll around until the afternoon in your favorite pajamas, an oversized bathrobe, some colorful socks, and slippers.

154

Heed your heart as well as your head.

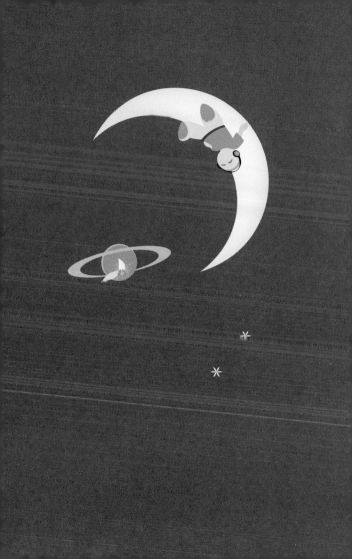

Sylvia Boorstein

"Don't just do something. Sit there."

Create a collage.

158

Every evening, list five things
that happened that day for which
you are grateful.

"HAVE NOTHING IN YOUR HOUSES THAT
YOU DO NOT KNOW TO BE USEFUL,
OR BELIEVE TO BE BEAUTIFUL."

William Morris

Take a trip to a museum, arboretum, or planetarium. Sign up for a walking tour of neighborhood architectural styles. Try something new or rekindle an old interest.

161

Lie flat on your back on a soft surface with your legs on the floor and your feet 6 to 8 inches apart. Place your hands by your sides, palms up. Take slow, deep breaths. Release your tension into the ground.

162

"A SPIRITUAL RETREAT IS MEDICINE FOR
SOUL STARVATION. THE RETREAT IS NOT
AN END IN ITSELF; IT IS SIMPLY A METHOD
TO HELP US SLOW DOWN AND STOP.
THROUGH SILENCE, SOLITARY PRACTICE,
AND SIMPLE LIVING, WE BEGIN TO FILL
THE EMPTY RESERVOIR."

David A. Cooper

163

Sew or purchase an herbal sleep pillow
made to fit between your pillowcase
and pillow.

Consider an inexpensive getaway.

Anything worth doing
is worth doing

S

L

SPEED LIMIT 10

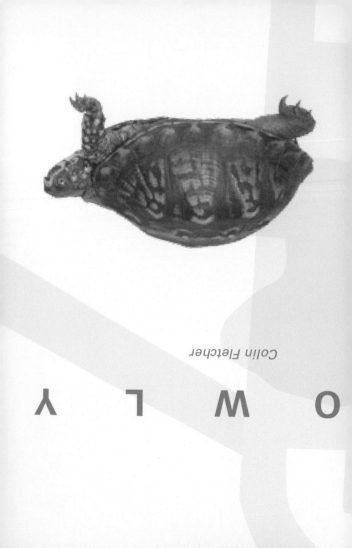

OWLY

Colin Fletcher

Imagine yourself in a field of wildflowers.

Skip a Slinky down the stairs, "walk the dog" with a yo-yo, or count the times you can hit the ball on its attached wooden paddle.

Stroll through a greenhouse and you'll flourish right along with the flowers.

Enjoy community entertainment
at a street fair or festival.

"WHEN WE FIND OUR RHYTHM OF
COMPASSION WE HAVE COME HOME, WE
ARE IN A STATE OF GRACE. WE ARE IN
TUNE WITH A GREAT UNIVERSAL CADENCE
WHERE A RICH INNER LIFE IS EXQUISITELY
BALANCED WITH A PASSIONATE ENGAGE-
MENT WITH THE WORLD."

Gail Straub

172

Be here now.

Sit by the water's edge. Skip stones across a pond. Dip your toes in the lake. Listen to the surf break.

Romantic fantasies lessen pain
and promote relaxation.

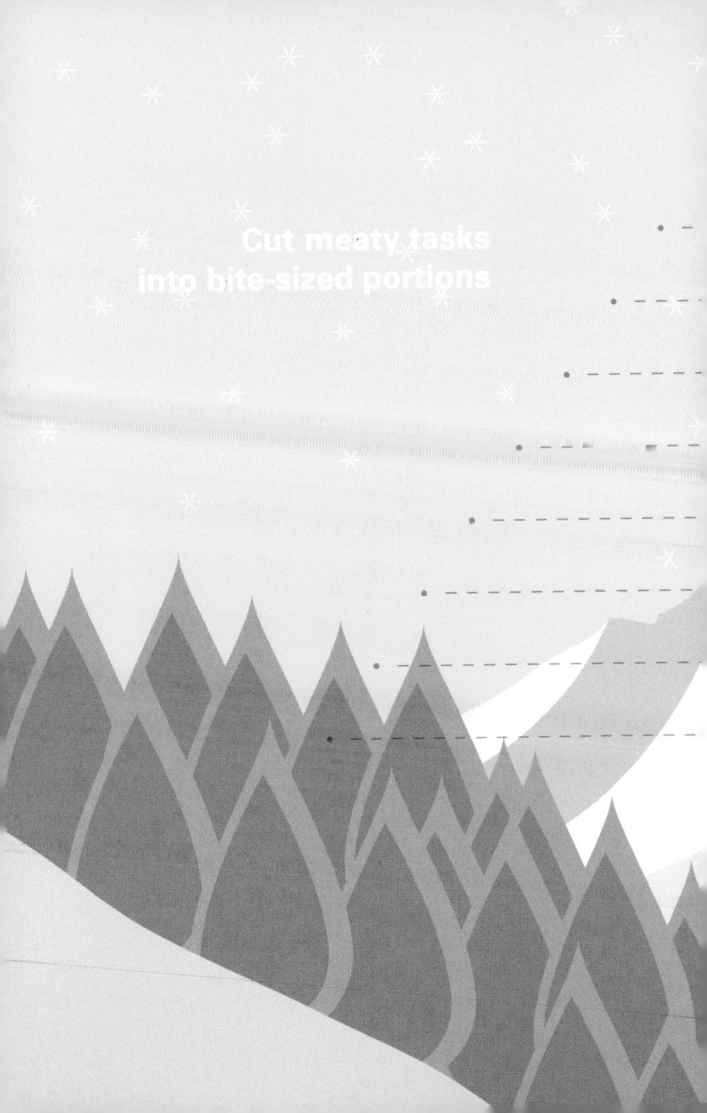

Cut meaty tasks
into bite-sized portions

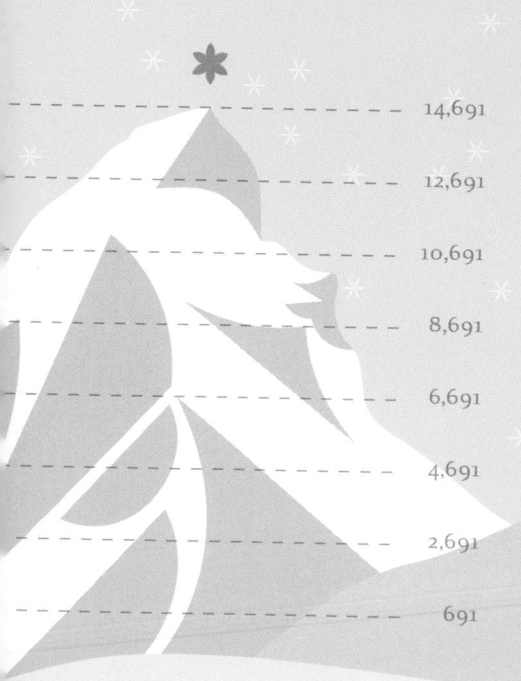

14,691

12,691

10,691

8,691

6,691

4,691

2,691

691

Stop doing and start being. Today, see how long you can do nothing.

Close a day of active outdoor activity with star watching and singing around the campfire.

179

Daydreaming is not a waste of time.

Go for a Sunday drive. Cruise the countryside, stopping at farm stands and flea markets.

For a melodic meditation, musicians recommend performing an old favorite piece rather than a new challenging one.

Social connections strengthen your mind, body, and spirit.

Go outdoors and play catch or bounce, hop, and roll on inflatable jumbo gym balls.

"LIFE IS A GOOD TEACHER
AND A GOOD FRIEND."

Pema Chodron

teaches us how to quiet
our overactive brains

and experience a
sense of serenity.

Napping in advance of a long stretch
of activity can improve one's memory,
mood, judgment, and creativity.

Take time to converse meaningfully
and touch gently.

Reserve a few hours a week for quiet reflection, meditation, or sharing a meal with others.

Find a new hobby.

"MEDITATION CAN RELEASE CERTAIN
FACETS OF YOUR MIND THAT USUALLY
REMAIN IN THE BACKGROUND. THEY
RESIDE IN EVERY PERSON'S MIND BUT
THEY COME OUT ONLY WHEN THEY
ARE WELCOMED WITH QUIETNESS,
AWARENESS, AND OBSERVATION.
THEY ARE CREATIVITY AND INTUITION."

American Yoga Association

192

When traveling, stash a small
herb-filled sachet in your carry-on
luggage to soothe you.

Peel an orange slowly and deliberately.
Let the aroma transport you.

Whistle a happy tune.

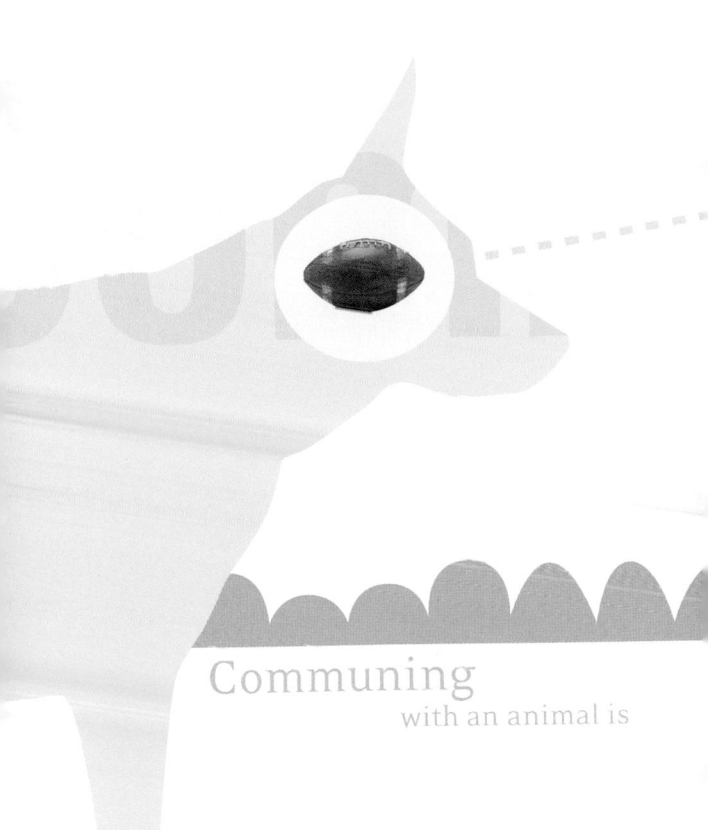

Communing
with an animal is

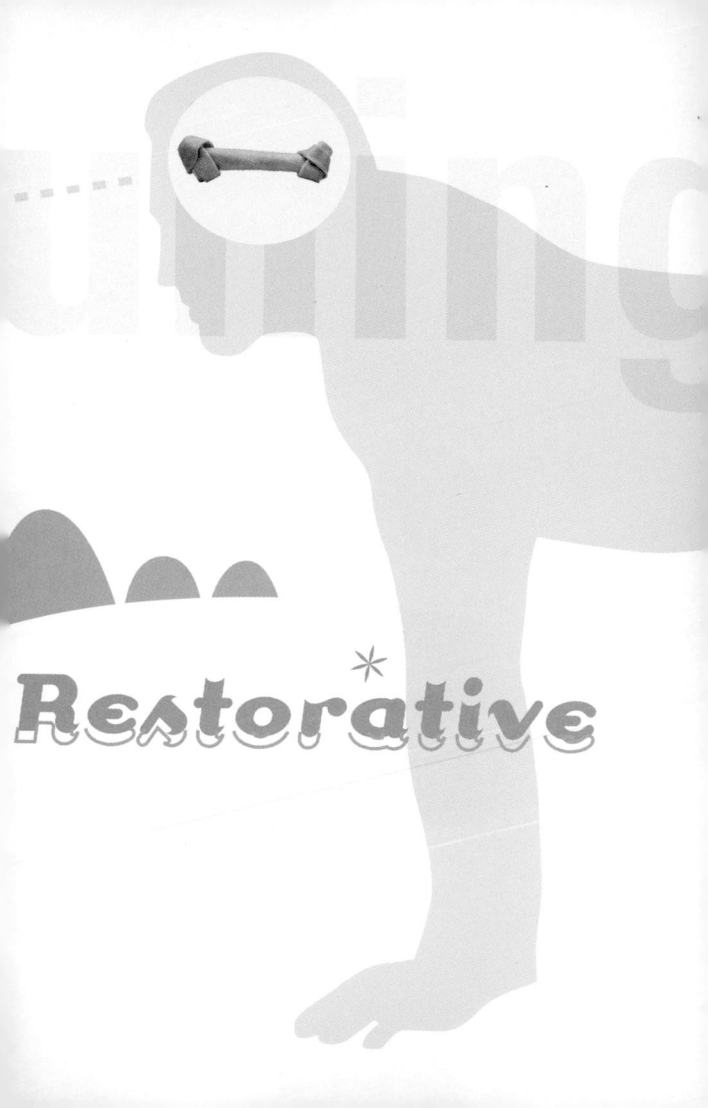

Restorative

Make snow angels.

"THE PRESENT MOMENT IS WHERE LIFE CAN BE FOUND, AND IF YOU DON'T ARRIVE THERE, YOU MISS YOUR APPOINTMENT WITH LIFE. YOU DON'T HAVE TO RUN ANYMORE. BREATHING IN, WE SAY, 'I HAVE ARRIVED.' BREATHING OUT, WE SAY, 'I AM HOME.'"

Thich Nhat Hanh

199

Heed the message "Mending is better than ending."

Take a stroll without a purpose
or a destination.

"THE WINDOW TO THE SPIRIT IS THE SILENT
SPACES BETWEEN OUR THOUGHTS."

Deepak Chopra

202

Be generous with your comfort and
support of others.

Avoid those last-minute trips to the store by purchasing duplicates of the items that you use frequently.

Fill a file with copies of thank you notes, moving tributes, honors, and awards that you've received. Reread this pile of special missives when skies are gray.

Writing by hand gives you a chance to reflect.

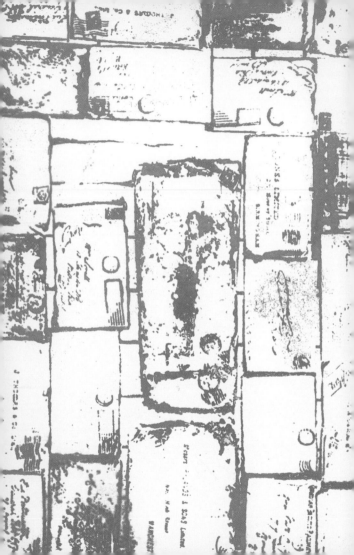

Let your cares float away during a day spent sailing or canoeing on the water.

Leaf through a photo album for a close-up of your past.

Chamomile tea, served hot or chilled, is a mild-tasting, wonderfully relaxing beverage.

"PEOPLE WHO HAVE A LOT OF MONEY
AND NO TIME WE CALL 'RICH.' PEOPLE
WHO HAVE TIME BUT NO MONEY WE
CALL 'POOR.' YET THE MOST PRECIOUS
GIFTS — LOVE, FRIENDSHIP, TIME WITH
LOVED ONES — GROW ONLY IN THE
SWEET SOIL OF 'UNPRODUCTIVE' TIME."

Wayne Muller

211

Design a personal pilgrimage for internal peace.

Listen for the voice
of your inner wisdom.

Don't jump out of bed. Open your eyes, slowly uncurl, and savor the state of mind between dreaming and alertness. Stretch and smile.

Be technology-free for one day.

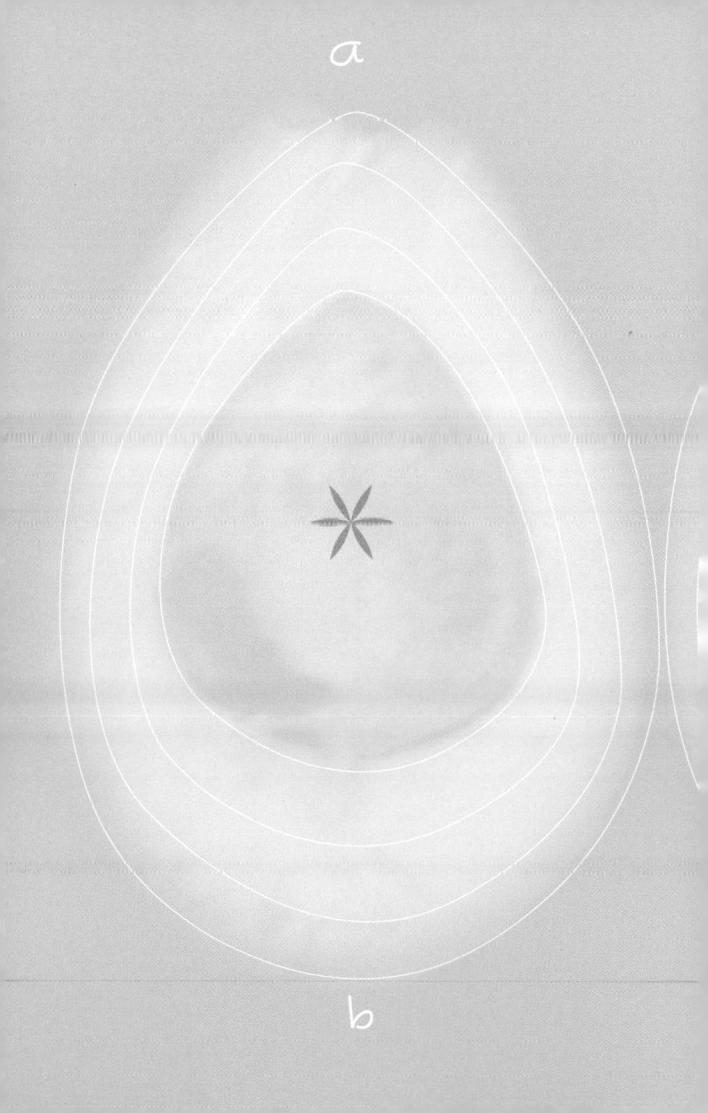

b

"WHEN ONE IS A STRANGER
TO ONESELF, THEN ONE IS   ESTRANGED
FROM OTHERS, TOO. ONLY WHEN ONE
IS CONNECTED TO ONE'S CORE IS ONE
CONNECTED TO OTHERS. THE CORE,
THE INNER SPRING, CAN BEST BE FOUND
THROUGH   SOLITUDE."

Anne Morrow Lindbergh

a

Reserve one evening a week to leisurely
enjoy a traditional meal.

Hum a lullaby to a little one
while swaying in a rocking chair.

"WE NEED TIME TO DREAM, TIME TO
REMEMBER, AND TIME TO REACH
THE INFINITE, TIME TO BE."

Gladys Taber

220

Shop at the farmers' market. This true soul food will nourish your body and your spirit.

222

Everyone needs a good cry.

Think of the telephone as a bell sounding the call for inner balance. Take deep and slow breaths while you wait until the second or third ring to pick up.

223

Seek wisdom in the open air.

Rainbow searching is both an art
and a science.

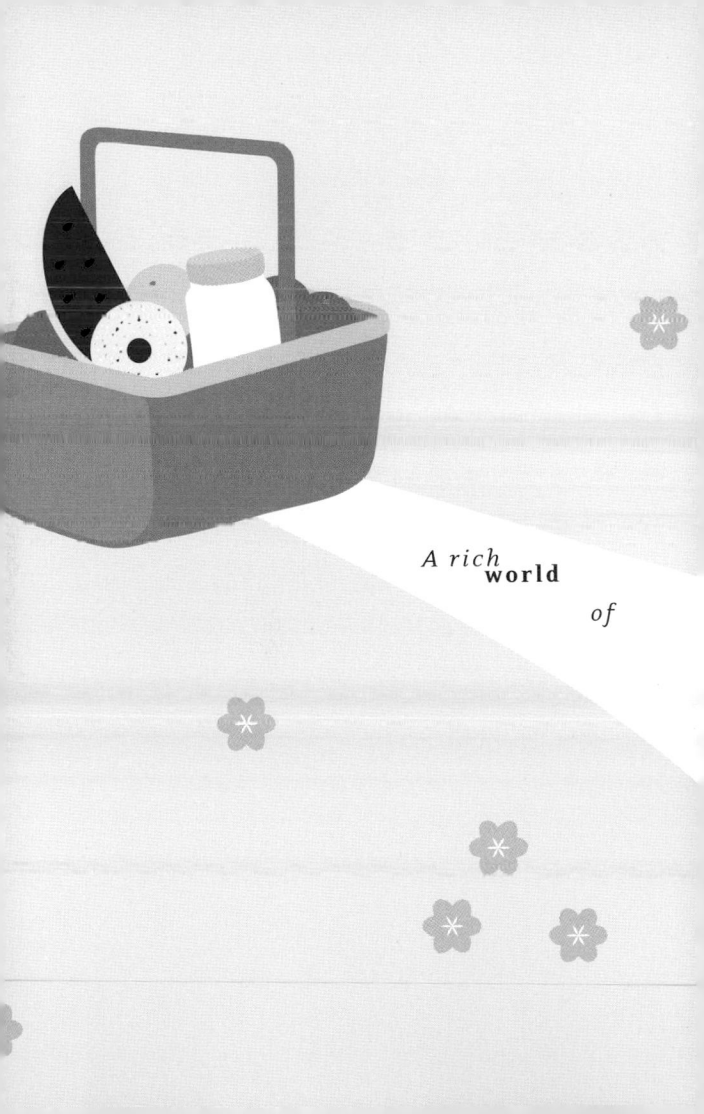

A rich **world** *of*

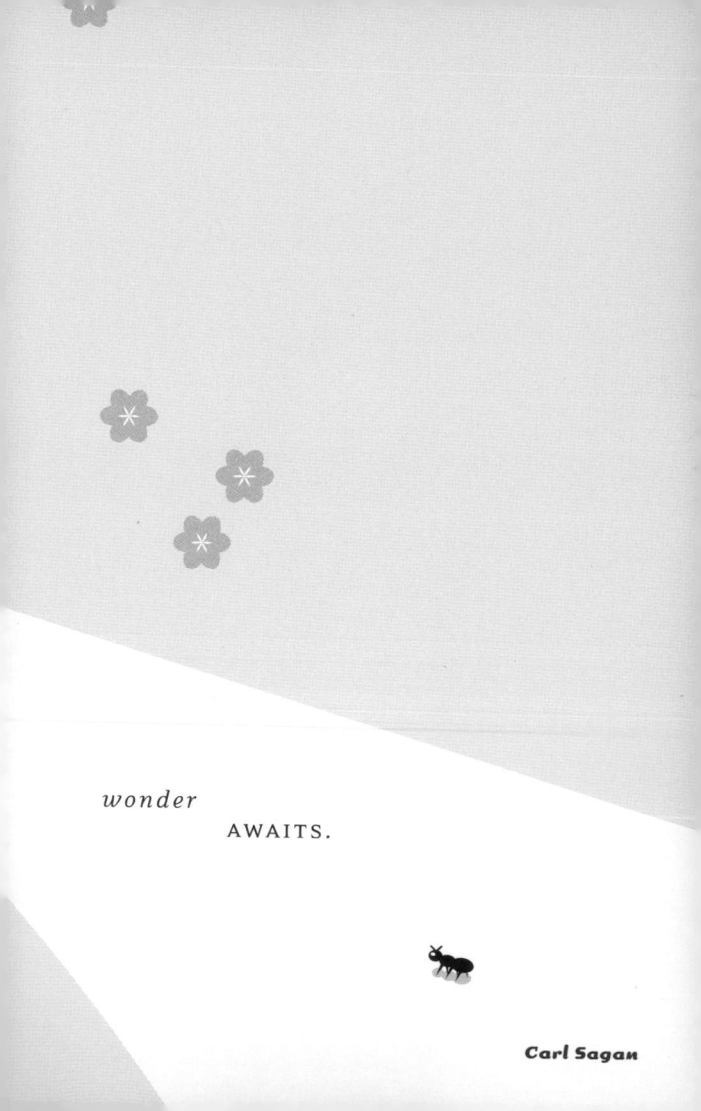

wonder
AWAITS.

Carl Sagan

Provide a physical outlet for anger and frustration.

228

Avoid unnecessary meetings, cancel unimportant commitments, screen phone calls, and limit time spent responding to e-mail and other messages.

Juggling unravels jangled nerves.
If you stick with it, you will also
develop a meditative concentration.

Go to the playground and kid around
on the swings, slide, and seesaw.

When stressed, silently count backward from 100 by sevens.

Stand your ground.

Appreciate your own achievements.

234

235

Grace your house with
a symbol of serenity.

LIFT ME UP